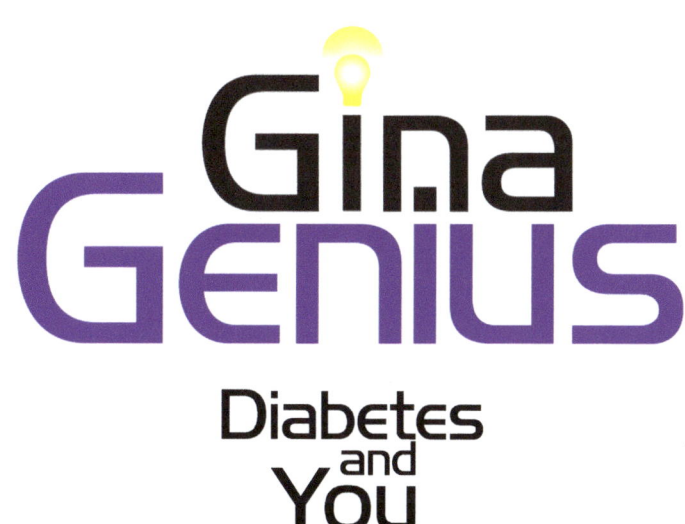

Gina Genius

Diabetes and You

Created by Meghan Kube

Summary: Gina Genius is actually a genius! She enjoys teaching other children about anything and everything she can!

All information within this text is researched through sources online and obtained through personal experience. Sources sited.

I would like to thank my family and friends who have helped me throughout my journey of living with diabetes.

I would also like to thank my diabetes educators and doctors that helped me learn how to manage my life with diabetes.

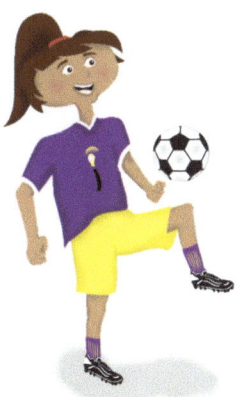

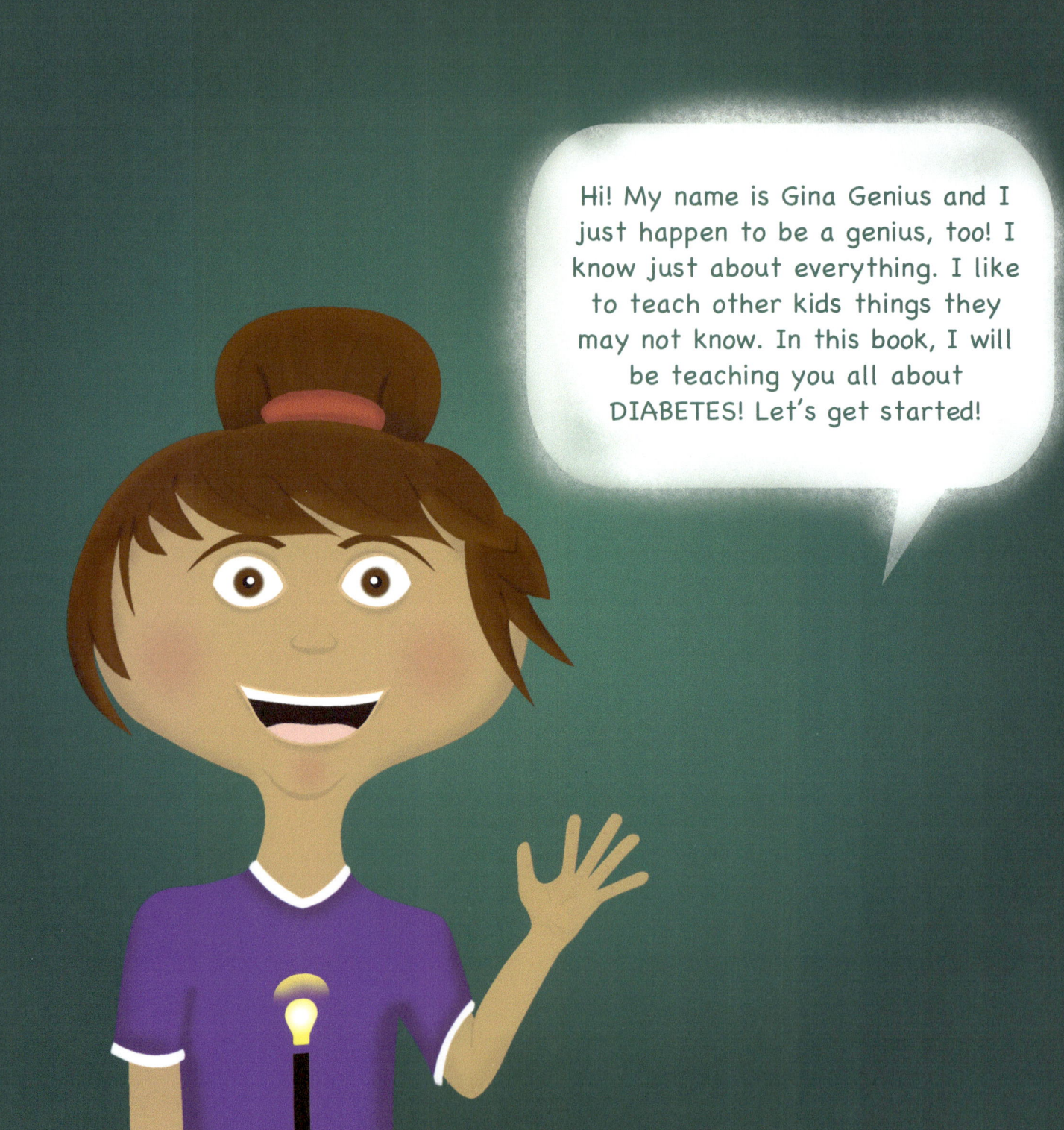

Diabetes
and
You

Diabetes is a disease in which the body produces little to no insulin that can cause blood glucose, or blood sugar, to rise and fall. It's important to know what it is and how it works so that you can stay healthy. I can teach you what diabetes is, how it works, and if you are diabetic just like me, how to take care of yourself.

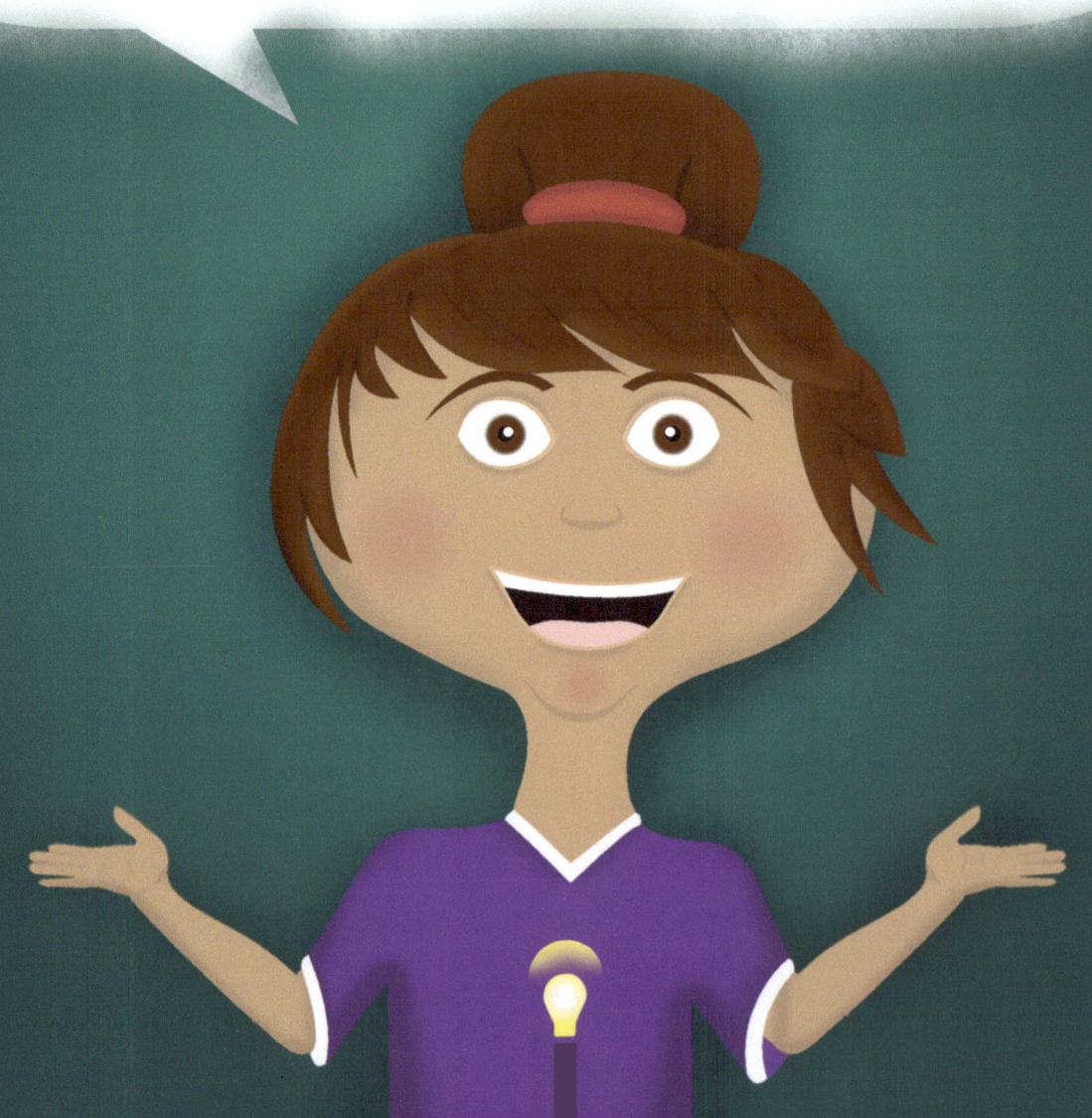

What is Diabetes?

29 million Americans are diagnosed with diabetes.
That's about 1 in every 10 Americans.

Diabetes can be controlled with the help of...

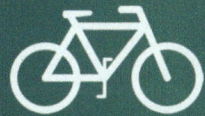

Exercise + Diet

Exercise requires energy and burns up sugar. A healthy style choice of food can make a big difference in controlling diabetes.

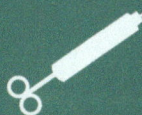

Insulin

Insulin helps use up the glucose in the bloodstream.

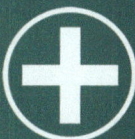

Doctors

Doctors can help you plan a routine to help manage diabetes.

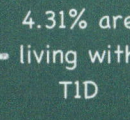

4.31% are living with T1D

95.69% are living with Pre-diabetes or T2D

2 Types

Type 1 (T1D) - the body requires the use of insulin to survive.

Type 2 (T2D) - the body may produce insulin, but not as well, and can be managed or even reversed with strict diet and healthy choices.

2

Healthy Lifestyle Choice

The most common question people have for diabetics is:

What do you eat?

So what does a diabetic's diet consist of?

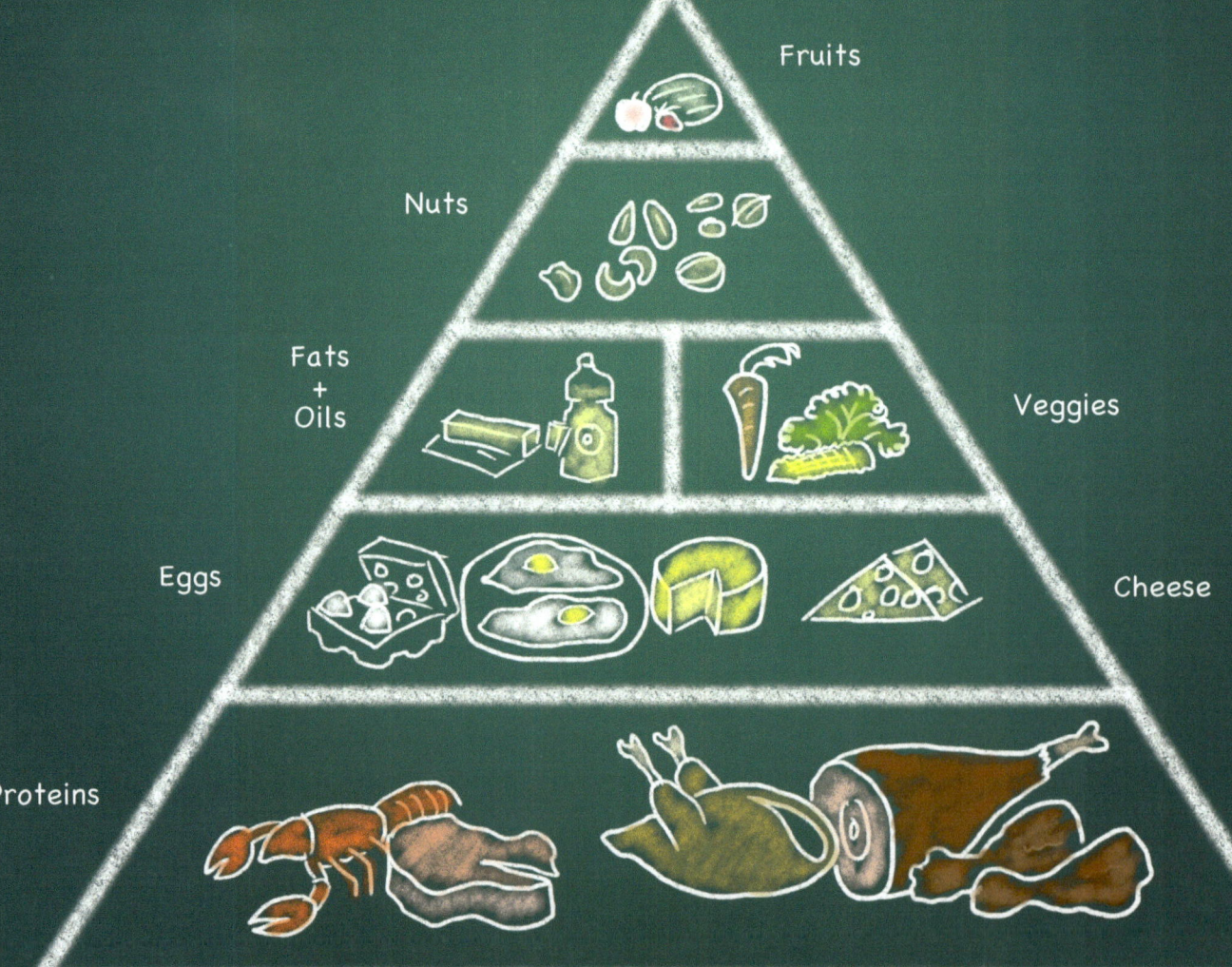

Fruits

Nuts

Fats + Oils

Veggies

Eggs

Cheese

Proteins

Here, we see a food chart specifically designed for diabetics to help control their blood sugar. There are foods that have a low carbohydrate count which is great for diabetics. The low carb count means that there will be less sugar in your blood. You can find the amount of carbs by looking at TOTAL CARBOHYDRATES in the nutrition facts.

From the chart, we can see that PROTEINS, EGGS, and CHEESES make up a large amount of the diet. As we go up in the pyramid, there are smaller portions as to which food group you should consume.

Of course it's not to say you can't have it, just not in large amounts. You can find more examples of what to eat and what to stay away from online or from your doctors.

Good vs Bad

Good
✓ Broccoli
✓ Whole Grains
✓ Sweet Potatoes
✓ Carrots
✓ Beans
✓ Spinach
✓ Mushrooms
✓ Cauliflower
✓ Apples, Oranges, etc

Bad
✓ White Bread
✓ Cereals
✓ Canned Veggies
✓ Canned Fruit
✓ Candied Fruit
✓ Fruit Juice

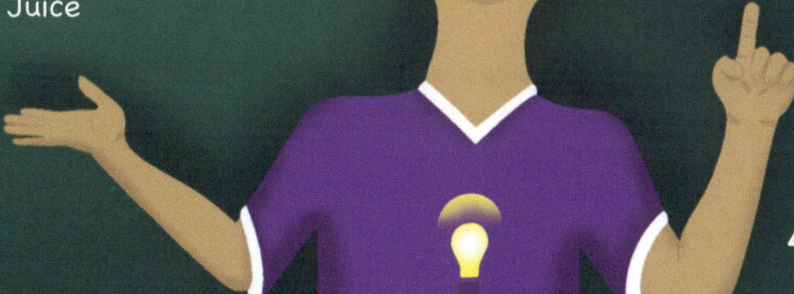

No Sugar Coating Here!

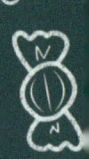

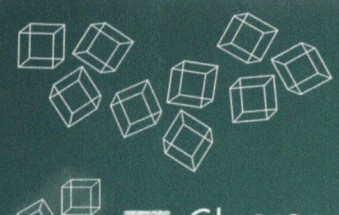

= Glucose

Just like cars need gas to run, we need glucose to operate

What is Glucose?

Glucose is a type of sugar your cells use for energy. Energy is needed for things like movement and even body functions.

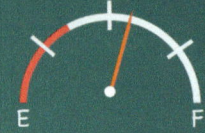

Our bodies need a steady amount of glucose to keep running. Diabetes makes it more difficult for the body to keep the blood sugar in a good range.

Where does it come from?

FOOD!

Most foods may have carbohydrates, a scientific term for sugar, or starch. Food is broken down into nutrients, like glucose, by digestion. Then it makes its way into your bloodstream.

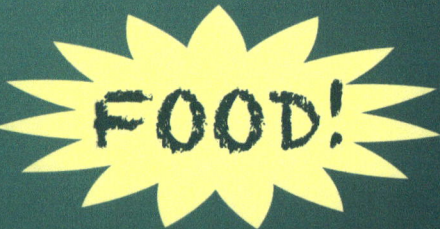

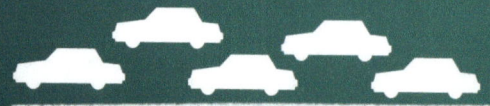

Traffic Jam!

The bloodstream acts just like a transportation system and takes the glucose throughout the body so that you can have energy. However, the body cannot use that energy without the help of insulin

Isn't it amazing what our bodies can do? When I go to my soccer games, I always bring something to snack on!

Which of these foods should I eat during soccer practice?

A. Fruits and Water
B. Cookies and Milk
C. Fast Food and Soda

Answer: A Fruits and Water

My Pancreas is just lazy.

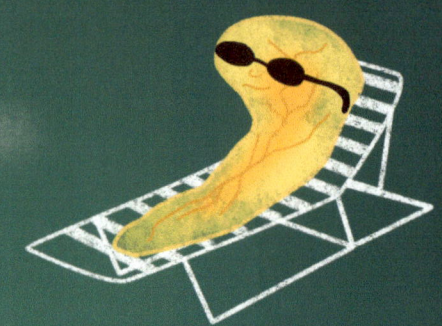

What is the Pancreas?

The pancreas is an organ that produces two types of hormones to balance your blood sugar. A person with diabetes produces little to none of these hormones.

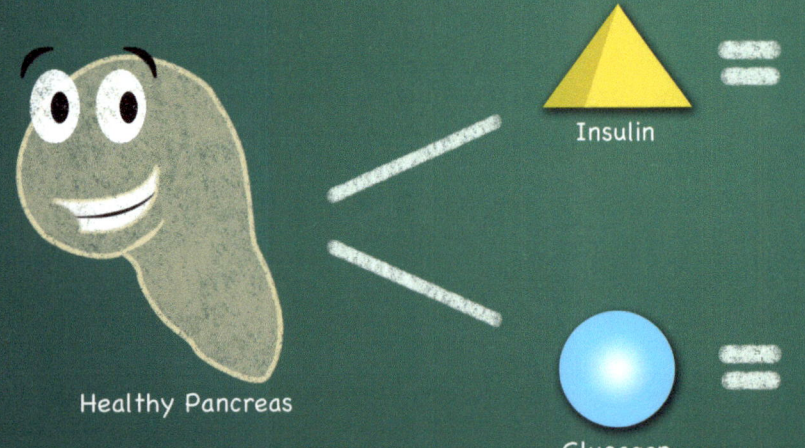

Insulin

Glucagon

Healthy Pancreas

Insulin is one of the hormones produced by the pancreas. Insulin's job is to move glucose into the cells for energy. It attaches to the outer wall of cells creating a chemical reaction. That's one of the reasons it's called the "key".

Glucagon is the second hormone that the pancreas produces. When the body does not have enough energy, the glucagon's job is to raise your blood sugar. Glucagon tells the liver to release the extra glucose into the bloodstream.

Skin

Bloodstream

Glucose

Cell

Insulin

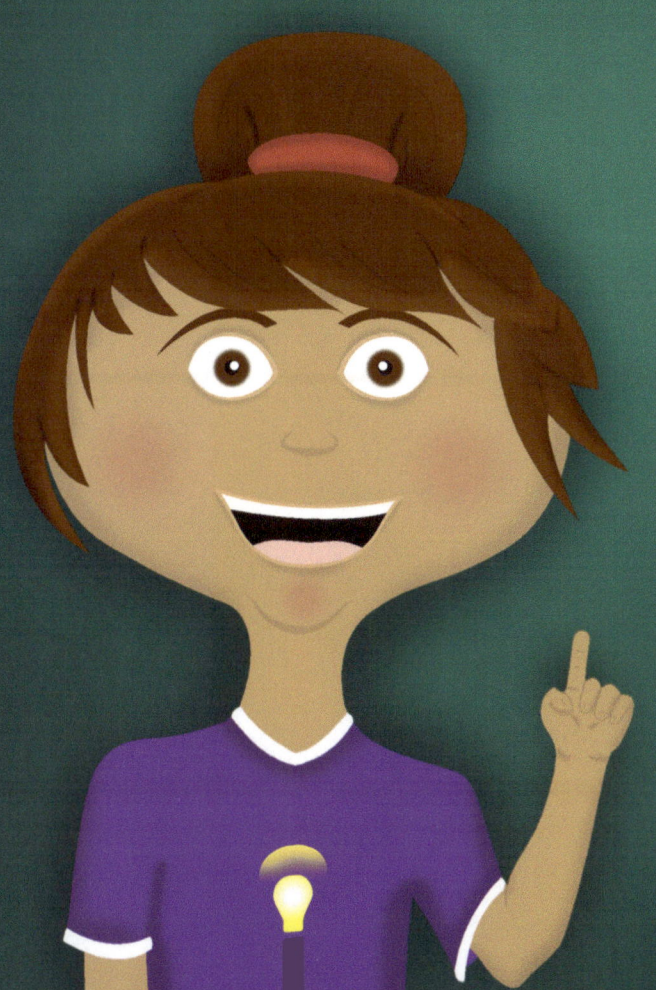

So far we've introduced WHAT diabetes is and HOW it works. Let's take a minute to see what you learned.

1. What does the body need in order to use glucose for energy?

      A. Sugar
      B. Insulin
      C. Water

2. What is the organ that produces insulin?

      A. Pancreas
      B. Liver
      C. Heart

3. Where does glucose, or sugar, come from?

      A. The Gas Station
      B. Water
      C. Food

4. What is glucagon's job?

      A. To raise blood sugar
      B. To cause a traffic jam
      C. To lower blood sugar

Answers: 1. B 2. A 3. C 4. A

Great! I hope you are learning as much as I am! You can never know too much! Now that we've introduced diabetes, let's move on. A person with diabetes will most likely need the help of insulin. One thing you need to know is the difference between basal and bolus.

Basal and Bolus

These are measurements of doses of insulin throughout your day. You take different amounts at certain times of the day

Two of a Kind

Basal

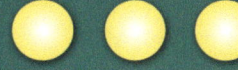

Basal Insulin

Basal insulin is small amounts of insulin
needed for small amounts of glucose.
Usually between meals or while you sleep.

Bolus

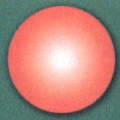

Bolus Insulin

Bolus insulin is larger amounts of insulin
needed for bigger amounts of glucose in
the bloodstream, like when you eat.

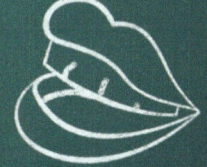

Timeline Example

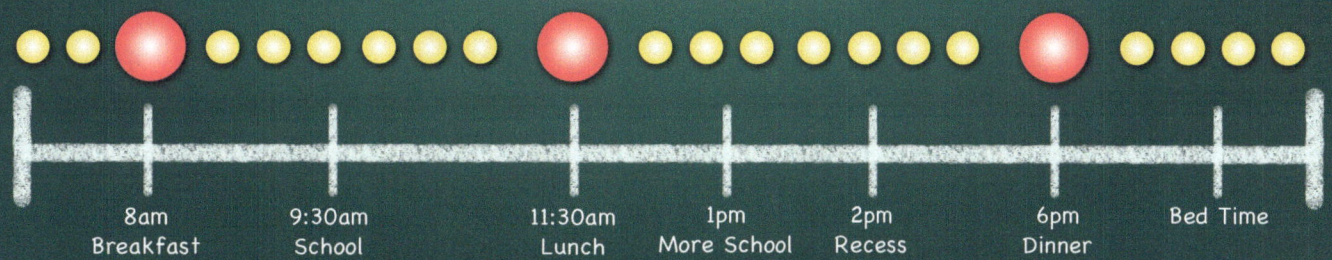

| 8am | 9:30am | 11:30am | 1pm | 2pm | 6pm | Bed Time |
| Breakfast | School | Lunch | More School | Recess | Dinner | |

There are a few ways for someone with diabetes to manage it. There are options for everyone! It all depends on what works for you best. With the help of endocrinologists and educators, you can make a decision on which method you prefer.

Endocrinology

[en-doh-kruh-nol-uh-jee]

An endocrinologist is someone who studies the endocrine system. Endocrinology is the study of a system of glands that spread hormones throughout the body. One of those glands is the pancreas. Your primary doctor can recommend an endocrinologist for you to gain the best treatment.

The Managers

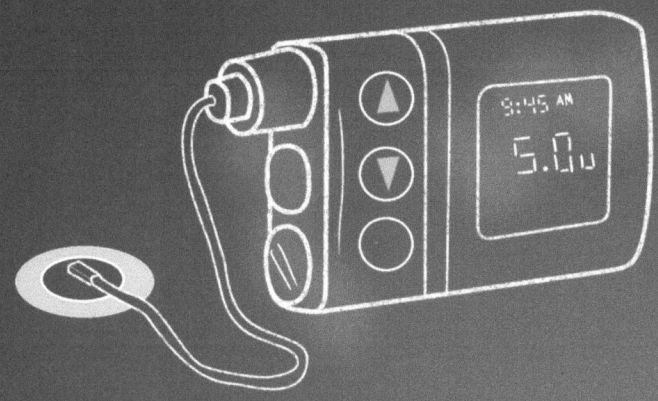

The Insulin Pump

Insulin pumps can deliver insulin in increments as small as 0.125 units giving you great control over your diabetes.

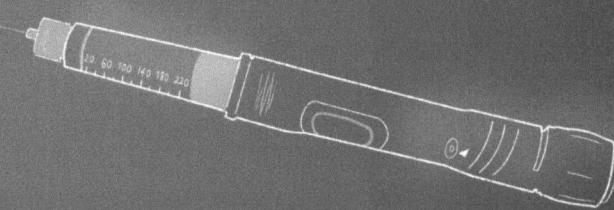

The Insulin Pen

While using insulin pens to control diabetes, there are two that are needed. One pen for a long acting insulin (basal) and one pen for fast acting insulin (bolus).

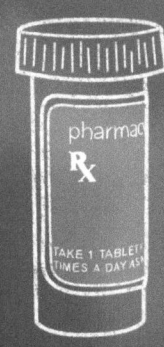

The Insulin Medicine

Some people can manage their diabetes with the use of medication through pills.

Finger Prickin' Good

What is Blood Sugar?

If you are diabetic, you will most likely carry a meter with you at all times. This little thing can tell you how much glucose you have in your bloodstream. It is measured as milligrams per deciliters (mg/dL). The ideal range is generally between 70 and 180.

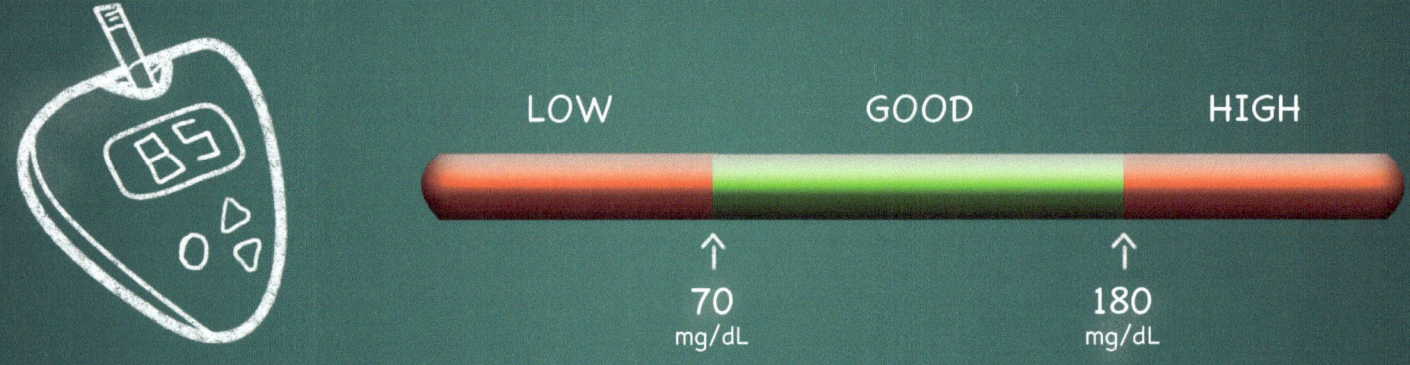

LOW   GOOD   HIGH

↑   ↑
70   180
mg/dL   mg/dL

Why is it important?

Monitoring your blood sugar can have several benefits. Keeping track of your blood sugar can help you take the correct dose of insulin as well as knowing what direction you are headed (high or low). In addition, keeping your sugar in a good range can help lower your A1C, a measurement of blood sugar over a larger amount of time, and improving your overall health.

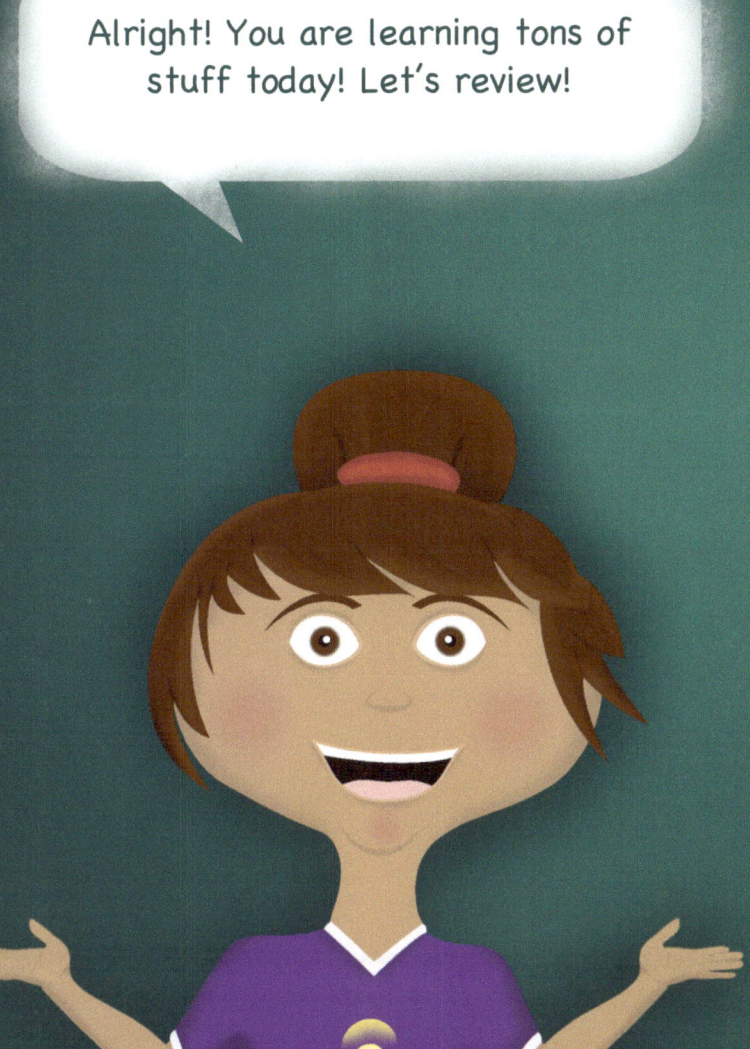

Alright! You are learning tons of stuff today! Let's review!

So far, we've learned:

- Basal insulin is the steady supply of insulin throughout the day

- Bolus insulin is for when you eat

- Endocrinologists are doctors who can help people with diabetes

- There are many ways to take insulin

- A glucose meter is used to monitor your blood sugar

- Checking blood sugar regularly can have long term health benefits

We are making great progress! Next, we'll learn about the best times to check your blood sugar as well as what to do when you are sick. Remember, the key to managing diabetes is to keep your sugar in check. Lastly, we'll go over the causes and symptoms of LOW and HIGH blood sugar. It's helpful to know the symptoms so that you may correct your blood sugar.

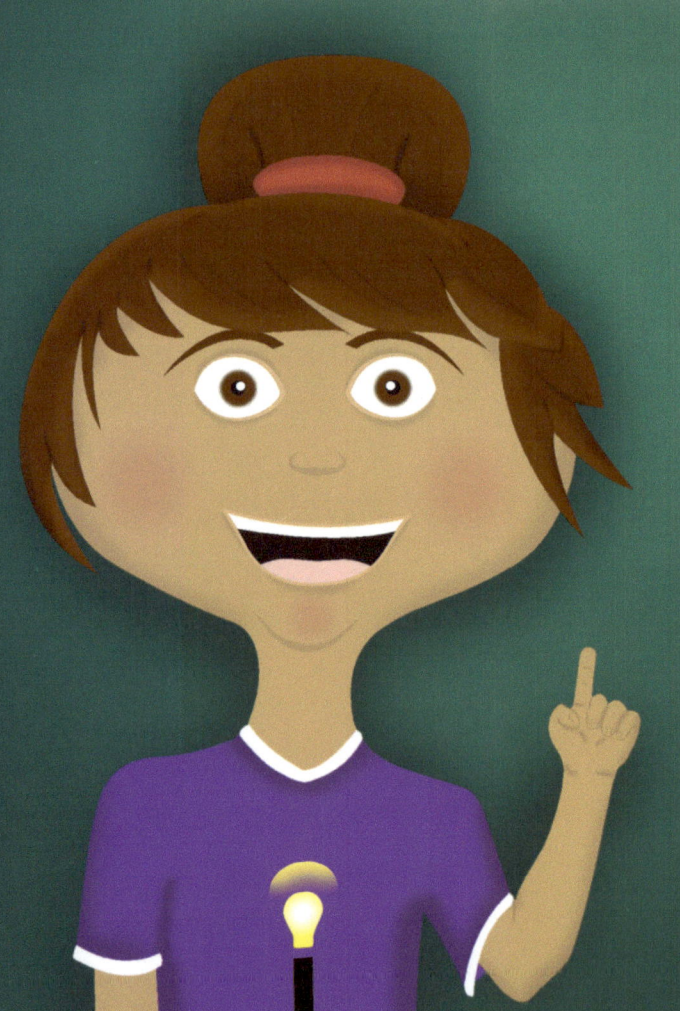

Check List

✓ When you wake up

✓ Before Breakfast

✓ Before Lunch

✓ Before Dinner

✓ Before Bed

Keep It In Check

When should your sugar be checked?

Checking your sugar regularly can help you monitor what direction you are heading; high or low. By monitoring it, your health will benefit in the long run.

You should check your sugar at least <u>4 times a day.</u>

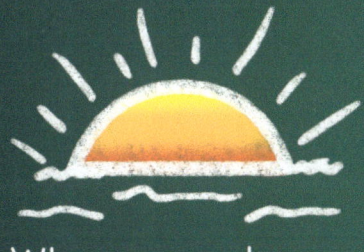

When you wake up

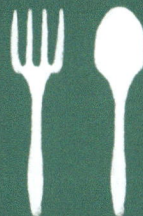

Before you eat breakfast, lunch, or dinner

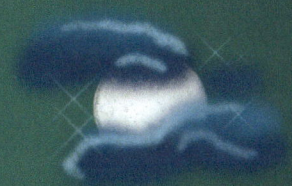

Before you go to sleep

What if you are sick?

If you are sick, your sugar may rise. But don't worry, just make sure that you:

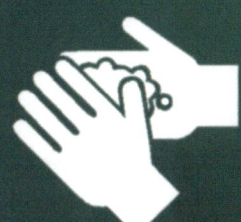

1. Keep your hands clean
2. Keep supplies clean
3. Check your sugar often
4. Check for ketones
5. Drink lots of fluids

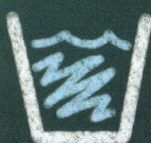

Helpful Hint: If you decide to take medicine, make sure to take a sugar-free or diabetic friendly medicine. You can ask a pharmacist for advice.

Don't Feel Down

What causes low blood sugar?

The two most common reasons of low blood sugar are:

1.  Exercise

2. 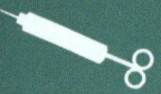 Too Much Insulin

Symptoms

Shaking

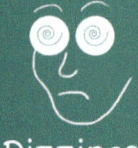
Dizziness

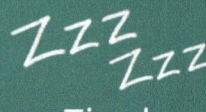
Tired

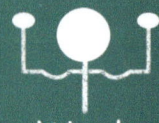
Weak

What to do:

1. Check your blood sugar
2. Eat or drink about 15g of carbs
3. Recheck after 15 minutes

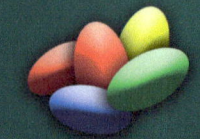
Jelly Beans

Severe Lows

For cases when blood sugar is extremely low there are Glucagon Emergency Kits.

Severe lows are possible and symptoms may not make appearances right away. In these cases, someone else may need to help you.

*Glucagon Emergency Kits can be obtained through prescription.

High Rise Acts

What causes high blood sugar?

The four most common reasons of high blood sugar are:

1. 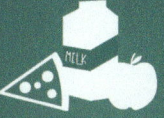 Not enough or weak insulin

2. 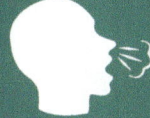 Too much food

3. 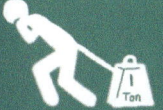 Illness or sickness

4. Stress

Symptoms

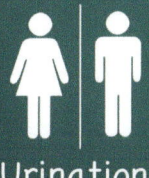 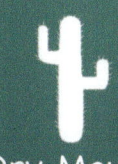  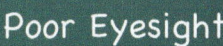 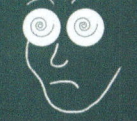

Urination   Dry Mouth   Tired   Poor Eyesight   Dizziness

What to do:

1. Check your blood sugar
2. Insulin correction
3. Exercise
4. Drink a lot of water

Multiple High Readings

If you have multiple high readings, you may need to check for ketones. Ketones are produced when the body is forced to use fat as its main source of energy. Ketones are acids that are very harmful for your body.

You can buy test strips at your local pharmacy

18

Well that's all I have on Diabetes! There is always tons more to learn. Let's go over the key points one last time!

Review

✓ Diabetes is a disease that affects blood sugar

✓ Insulin is necessary to control blood sugar levels

✓ Insulin is the "key" to the body using energy

✓ Glucose is the "fuel" for our bodies

1. The pancreas produces two hormones, glucagon and _____.
     A. Insulin
     B. Sugar
     C. Glucose

2. What are the two types of insulin?
     A. Bogus and Basal
     B. Basal and Bolus
     C. Glucagon and insulin

3. Monitoring your blood sugar regularly is good for your health.
     A. True
     B. False

4. You should check your sugar at least ___ times a day.
     A. 8
     B. 2
     C. 4

5. Circle all that apply. If you are sick, you should:
     A. Keep your hands clean
     B. Ignore your symptoms
     C. Check your blood sugar often
     D. Check for ketones
     E. Play outside

6. One cause of LOW blood sugar is?
     A. Too much food
     B. Not enough insulin
     C. Exercise

7. One cause of HIGH blood sugar is?
     A. Illness
     B. Too much insulin
     C. Not enough food

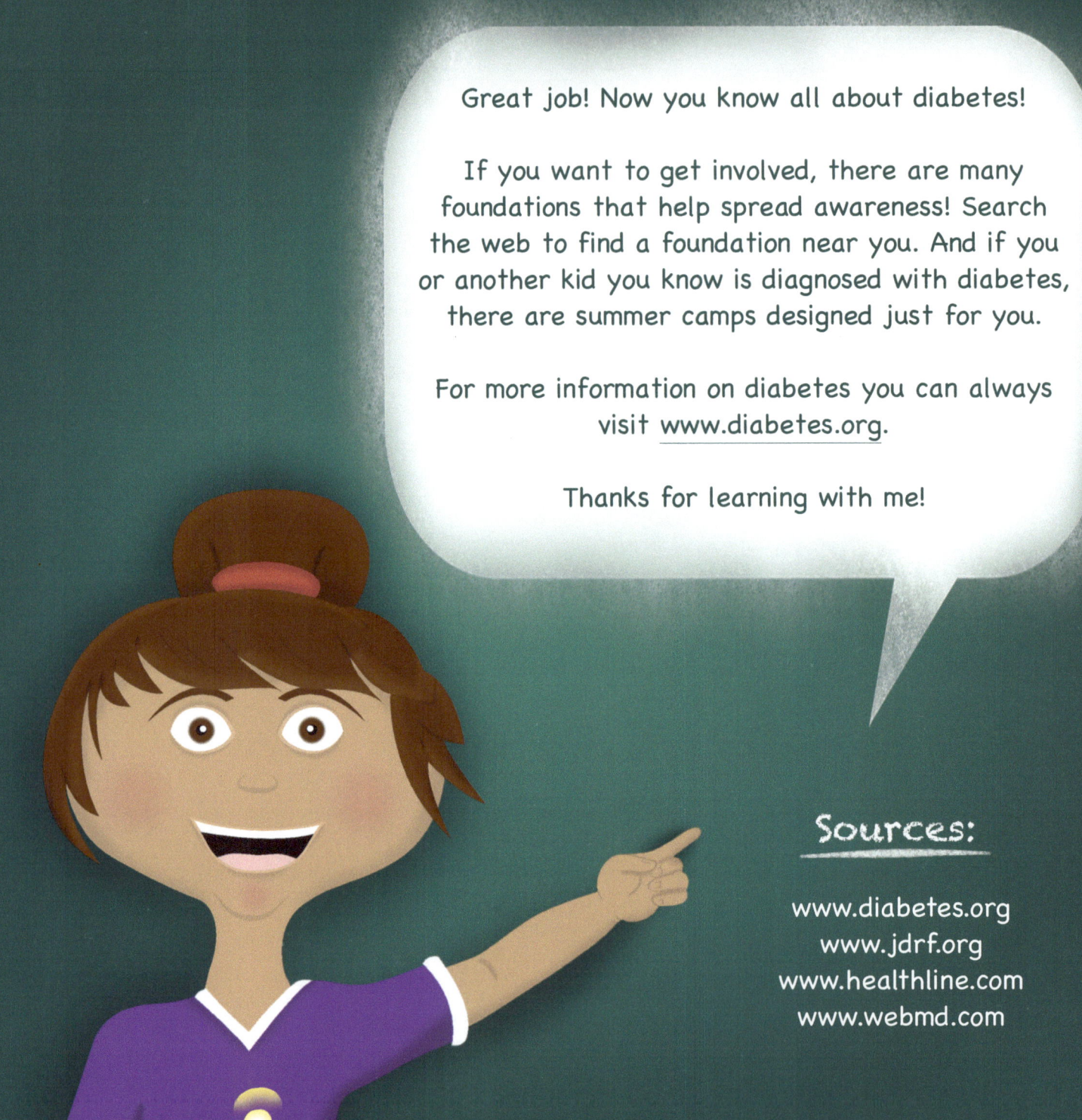

www.ingramcontent.com/pod-product-compliance
Lightning Source LLC
Chambersburg PA
CBHW040308010626
45792CB00025B/1695